GYMNASTICS:

The Round Off - Key to Advanced Tumbling

COACH RIK

Richardson Publishing, Inc.

GYMNASTICS: The Round Off - Key to Advanced Tumbling

COACH RIK

ISBN: 978-1-935683-14-8 (paperback)

Richardson Publishing, Inc.
PO Box 162115
Altamonte Springs, FL 32716
coachrik@aol.com

WARNING: Any activity, especially one with a high degree of motion, rotation, and height, (many times in an inverted (upside-down) position) carries with it a greater potential for injury than normal daily activity. Landing on the head or neck could cause serious and irreparable harm with the potential for fatal consequences to the individual. For this reason, it is advised / demanded that you seek training and supervision from Safety Certified gymnastics or cheer coach before using this material for any purpose.

Only a Safety Certified coach with professional membership in organizations such as USAG, USAIGC, AAU, YMCA and other recognized gymnastics associations should use this material. No skills should ever be practiced without proper and adequate gymnastics equipment under the supervision of a properly certified and professional gymnastics coach.

See "Specific Disclaimer" page 3.

Specific Disclaimer

The purpose of this book is to provide the reader with general information regarding the subject matter covered. Because every training, coaching, spotting, or competitive situation is different, and varies based on the need(s) of each gymnast, specific advice should be tailored to the particular needs and/or circumstances of each gymnast. For this reason, the reader is advised / required to consult with his or her own USAG Safety Certified Gymnastics Coach regarding each gymnast's specific training situation and physical, technical, and psychological training needs.

The author has taken every reasonable and prudent precaution in the preparation of this book and believes the facts presented in the book are accurate as of the date it was written. However, neither the author nor the publisher assumes any responsibility for any errors or omissions. The author and publisher specifically disclaim any liability resulting from the use or application of the information contained in this book, and the information is not intended to serve as legal, medical, or technical advice related to individual situations in the performance or training of gymnastics skills.

Because of the wide range of body shapes, technical awareness, physical preparation, and psychological readiness of each gymnast, it is imperative that all gymnastics skills be performed under the guidance of a qualified gymnastics coach (USAG Safety Certified) with the appropriate safety equipment and matting appropriate to the skill being performed.

Warning: The illustrations within this book are used to complement the text and are only approximations and are in no way the specific body positioning, starting / finishing poses, correct dance preparations, or appropriate positions for *every* gymnast due to the myriad sizes, shapes, and conditioning levels of any particular gymnast.

Basic Safety Guidelines

1. Gymnastics / tumbling is a fun activity, however, lack of focus during technical training, the performance of the skill, or in the workout area in general can lead to the potential of catastrophic injury. **Pay attention to your coach and the activity at hand.**

2. Use of any type of gymnastics, cheerleading, or tumbling equipment should only occur in the presence of qualified supervision.

3. Use appropriate progression techniques with regard to your physical conditioning, your knowledge of the timing, sequence, and specific attributes of the skill being performed, and the equipment necessary to each progression level.

4. In all training situations, proper matting, appropriate to the skill and progression level of the athlete should be used. Consult your coach.

5. Safe landing skills should be practiced for all tumbling skills and specifically for surfaces that are outside normal workout conditions.

6. **Always ask for a spot!** If you are ever in doubt about the safe performance of a tumbling skill, because of fear, lack of training, unusual conditions, or just a gut feeling – ask for a spot.

7. Responsibility for the performance of tumbling skills, and the potential for injury, outside the normal workout area and the guidelines listed here rests completely with the performer and the supervisor (parent, coach, director, etc.) of the activity.

8. In all instances, focus on preparing a safe environment for the performance of gymnastics / tumbling skills, which may include crowd control, hydration of athletes, shelter from the elements, and continuous checks of equipment to make sure it is in safe and acceptable working condition.

9. Prepare an "**Emergency Action Plan**" to implement in case of accident or injury.

10. **Always focus on Safety!**

Basic Body Positions

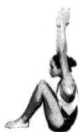

Tuck

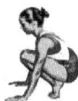

Squat

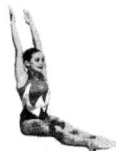

Pike

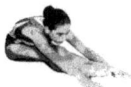

Closed Pike

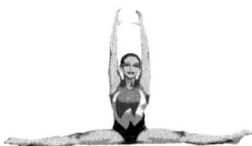

Straddle

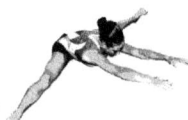

Closed Straddle

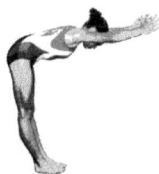

Pike Stand

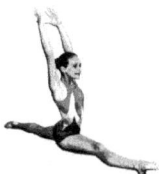

Forward Split

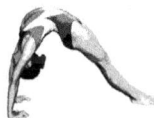

Bridge / Back Bend

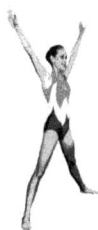

Straddle Stand

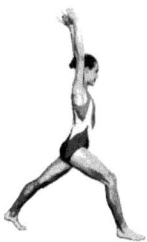

Lunge

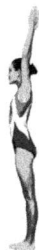

Stretch Position

Layout

Prone

Always focus on SAFETY!

Contents

Foreword

Safety is the first and main consideration when training any acrobatic or athletic skill – ALWAYS!

Any activity in life from taking a bath, playing basketball, even walking home after school carries varying degrees of risk for potential injury. An elbow in the face during a jump shot, a twisted ankle stepping off the curb, or a slip and fall getting out of the bathtub may cause serious injury. There is also the potential for significant injury when learning gymnastic, acrobatic, and tumbling skills.

The key to success for any athlete is patience, a desire to learn, and guidance from a qualified coach. Your desire to learn is obvious by the fact you are reading this book to learn and understand gymnastic techniques.

Note: The techniques presented are based on one "average" (in size, shape, and fitness level) athlete, which may be illustrated for some drills and techniques.

While the techniques presented may work adequately for this fictitious athlete, they may not work as well for the slightly overweight and less physically fit athlete. In addition, some athletes may need some preparatory work with strength training and nutrition.

Responsibility for the use and/or adaptation of these techniques is the sole responsibility of the individual using them.

The information contained in this guide provides a base level of knowledge about gymnastics, acrobatic, tumbling skills, and training techniques for the round off. Contact qualified coaches from a local gymnastics or cheer program to guide you in developing effective techniques specific to your needs to learn a round off, as well as providing spotting skills and training methods.

Note to Mom & Dad

Parents may listen in for information and ideas, but please defer to your coach's instructions regarding specific advice on your daughter's round off training.

When in doubt about any technique, always check with your local professional gymnastics and/or cheer coach for guidance.

Athletes get ready to start your engines!

My all-encompassing goal for this book is that you learn how to do a round off **SAFELY** while having **FUN** learning. That means there are no shortcuts.

Strength and flexibility will be the primary ingredient for your success in this endeavor, however, a safe environment (matting, spotters, etc.), an understanding of technique, and, of course, motivation are also important.

What I am trying to say is it will take focused effort on your part. There is no magic wand or special pixie dust to endow you with this skill. It has been said that "repetition is the mother of skill," and I believe that to be true, when you also add "feedback" to refine the skill, and "variety" to keep the whole process interesting and motivating.

It takes as long as it takes

I have not had the pleasure of meeting you in person so I can't determine your current level of fitness, your past background in acrobatics, gymnastics, or tumbling, or your current level of desire. I assume you have a high level of desire since you have purchased this book – thanks, by the way.

So, how long will it take to learn a correct round off?

It takes as long as it takes, and I do suggest that you take your time. You will refine the round off through hundreds of repetitions of drills and techniques. Long after you get your round off, you will review these skills time and again to continually refine your skill.

Throughout the whole process of learning a correct round off, I ask / desire / command you to focus on Safety (always), then fun, but certainly and without a doubt, I ask that you hold this one thought in your mind on every attempt: *"I **will do my best!"***

Athletes, raise your right hand
Repeat after me.

*"I do solemnly swear on my best pair of shoes and tightest jeans that I will read this book cover to cover and study every page **BEFORE** attempting any of the techniques, drills, or the round off itself."*

Introduction

Round Off: Key to Advanced Tumbling

Throwing yourself through the air on a wing and a prayer is the least effective method for doing a round off, especially if it leads into a back handspring or back somersault. Safety-wise, it is not an appropriate or helpful method of learning this skill.

Unfortunately, this method is all too common. Most often, what I see is an athlete running down the mat, then setting up the skill with a high hurdle and turning her body in the air as if she is doing a ½ on twist to the vault table. This early turn of the upper body usually results in a tumbling pass that swerves off the diagonal tumbling pass on a crooked path.

I want you to promise to learn the round off correctly. Not only will it make the back handspring easier to do; it will make it more powerful, and it will become a great lead-up skill for adding back somersaults. Sure, some of your friends will be bragging about their (*seizure technique*) round off back handsprings, but in the long run, if you put in the effort now, you will be a significantly better tumbler than the other athletes who cut corners.

"Where did little cartwheels and round offs come from, Coach Rik?"

Popular gymnastics mythology would seem to indicate that cartwheels came from ancient acrobats imitating the motions of a wheel on a cart, which had two boards crossing each other around which a wheel was placed.

The first cartwheels were completely sideways. Later, the cartwheel became stylized somewhat in that the tumbler may start from a forward-facing position, as though she was going to kick up to a handstand but at the last moment turned sideways to do a front to side cartwheel. Other times the tumbler started sideways but stepped down facing back the way she had come for a side to back cartwheel; still other tumblers combined all three positions and did front-side-back cartwheels. Eventually, and I am just guessing at this point, someone started a front side back cartwheel and accidentally finished with both feet together and the round off was born (*of course, I could be wrong*).

In any case, I am going to have you focus on learning a front-side-back cartwheel as the basis for a correct round off.

Front – Side – Back Cartwheels

Drill: Kick to (front) Handstand to & from a T-position.

Purpose: To teach you that driving your upper body down into a round off is like kicking into a handstand.

Directions: Starting in a stretch position on the floor, kick into a tight body handstand by moving through a T-position on the way up and as you step back down through an arabesque position to a stretch position.

(See Table of body positions on page 7.)

Handstand to & from a T-position.

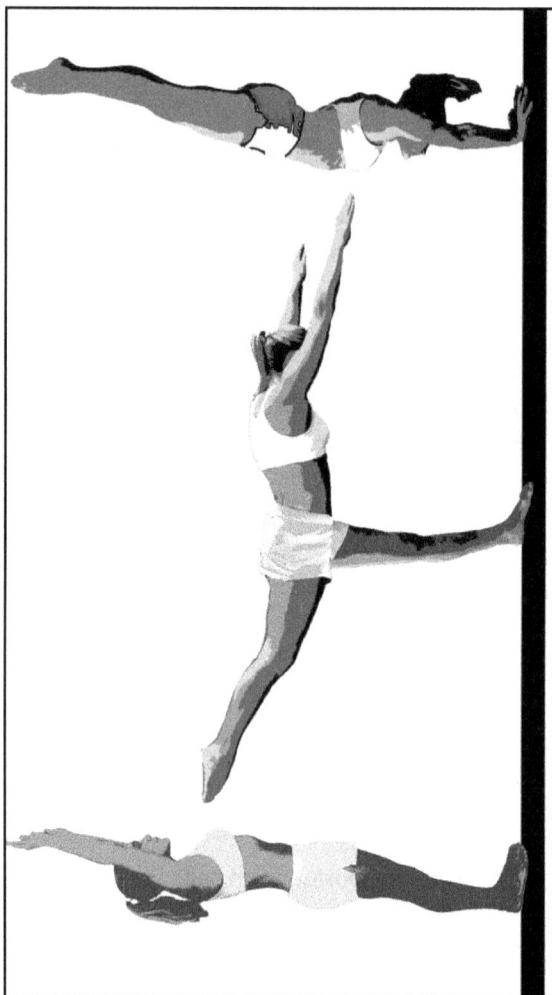

Drill: Side-to-side cartwheel [both sides]

Purpose: To develop control of the arms and legs while moving in a lateral or sideways movement pattern.

Set up: Place two or three 8" landing cushions up against the wall, securely fastened, so they don't fall down.

Directions: The objective is to do a cartwheel completely sideways – no turn out of the lead foot; keep your head in neutral (middle illustration incorrect); do not look in the direction of travel.

Side-to-side cartwheel

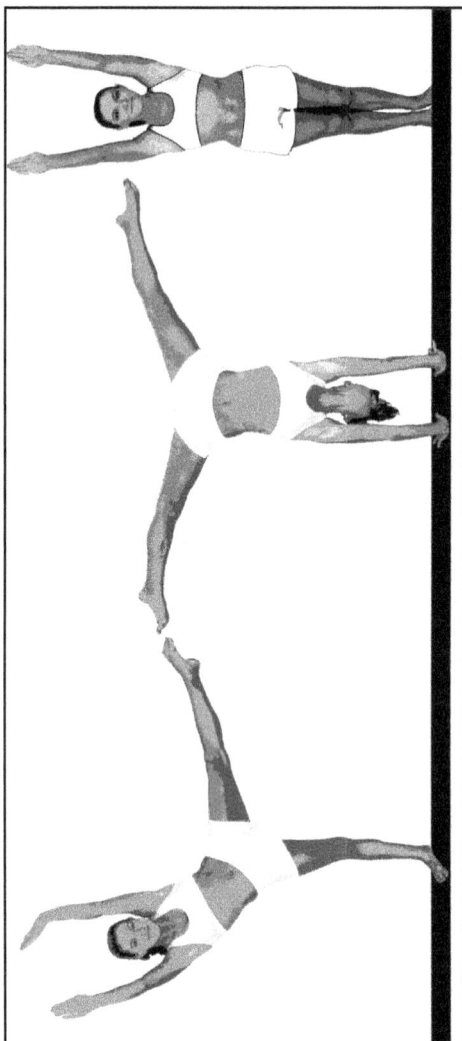

Canyon drill: (fun drill)

With the 8" landing mats against the wall (as described above) create a canyon by sliding a port-a-pit or stacks of panel mats that are higher than your waist. The idea is to do a completely sideways cartwheel in the canyon created without touching the mats on either side. After each turn, you will move the mats a little closer together.

You have mastered this skill when you can do a side-to-side cartwheel on the low beam.

Note: Remember to work this and all cartwheel drills to both right and left sides.

It may be more difficult on your non-dominant side (uncomfortable side) but it will help with bilateral symmetry and possibly open additional bridges between the right and left hemispheres of your brain through the corpus callosum. Don't worry about understanding this last paragraph; just pretend it's like vegetables, which are good for you. Eat your vegetables and do your cartwheels on both sides!

Drill: Side-to-side cartwheel, hold last leg at horizontal. [both sides]

Purpose: To teach you how to shift your weight from your upper body to your legs in a controlled manner.

Directions: The same as the side cartwheel except as the first foot steps down you will quickly lift the head and shoulders (staying sideways) until your weight is above your support leg and the opposite leg is held to the side in a horizontal position. It is important in this drill to keep the support leg straight and not allow the body to pivot. Practice this drill to both sides.

Side-to-side cartwheel, hold last leg at horizontal.

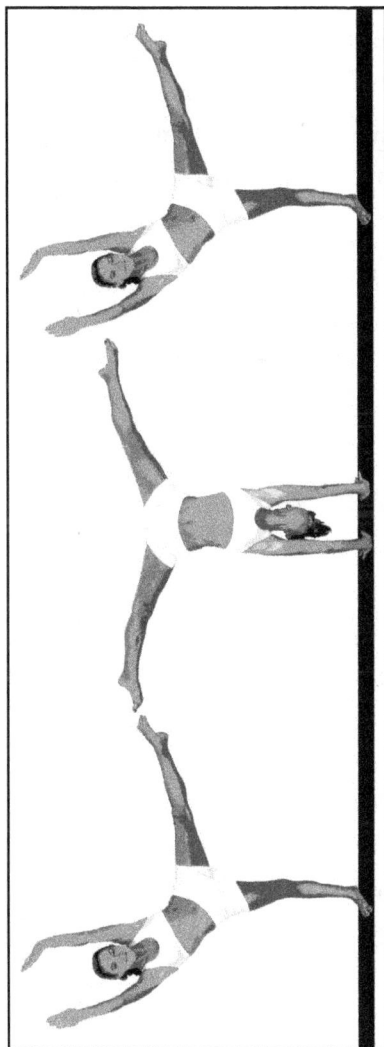

Drill: Front-to-side cartwheel, hold last leg up.

Purpose: To combine the "Front-to-Handstand," and "Side-to-Side," cartwheel drills.

Directions: The key to this drill is timing. You will kick up as though you are working on a handstand, however, when your fingertips are one inch from the floor you will quickly pivot your body sideways to finish as though you had done a side-to-side cartwheel [last leg held in horizontal position].

Front to side cartwheel hold last leg up

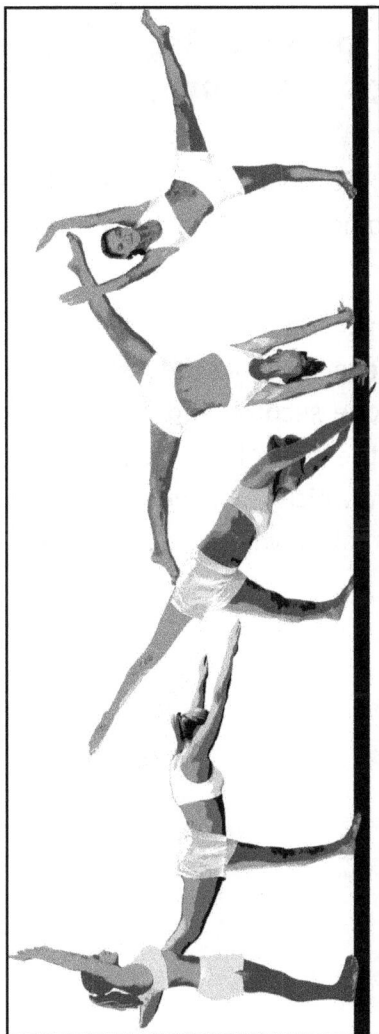

Drill: Front-to-side cartwheel, hold last leg in horizontal 1-second, and then pivot to backward finishing position pulling legs together and snapping chest upright.

Purpose: To help you focus on the final pivot as this will become the snap down portion of the round off.

Directions: Do a front-to-side cartwheel as described above and hold the last leg at the horizontal position for one second, and then pivot your body by rotating on the ball of your support leg foot in the direction from which you have come while snapping the leg at horizontal down and together with your support leg.

Front-to-side cartwheel, hold last leg in horizontal 1-second, and then pivot to backward finishing position.

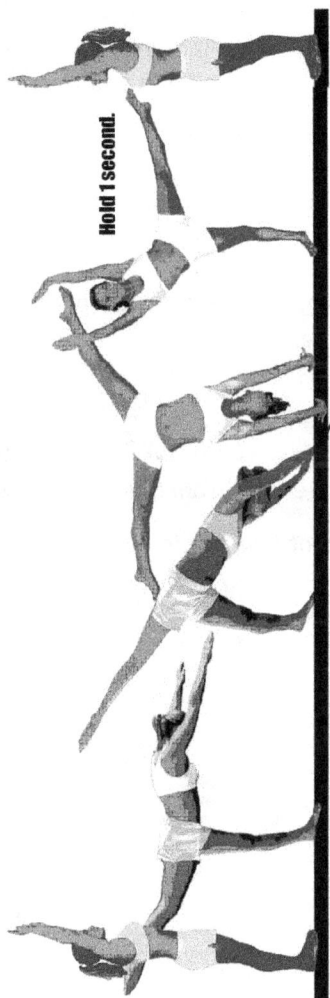

Hold 1 second.

Drill: Front-side-back cartwheel.

Purpose: This drill is the culmination of the above drills. It is important that each phase of this drill is distinctly shown. Allowing the front side of this drill to blur into the side portion because you turn too early (more than one inch above the floor) will cause you to develop bad habits.

Directions: The same as the above drill except there will be no pause or hold of the leg; you will move through the skill showing each position but continue to move smoothly to the end, which is a stretch position.

Special Note: Before the second leg closes with the support leg, the head, chest, and arms should already be up in the stretch position. If you have done the skill correctly, you will find that finishing in this position correctly develops some power and may cause you to take a step or two backwards to control the kinetic energy from the momentum of the skill.

You may notice that I am not including the "run, hurdle, RO" as a drill because I want you to focus on technique and get away from the erroneous thinking that a fast run is necessary.

Front-side-back cartwheel

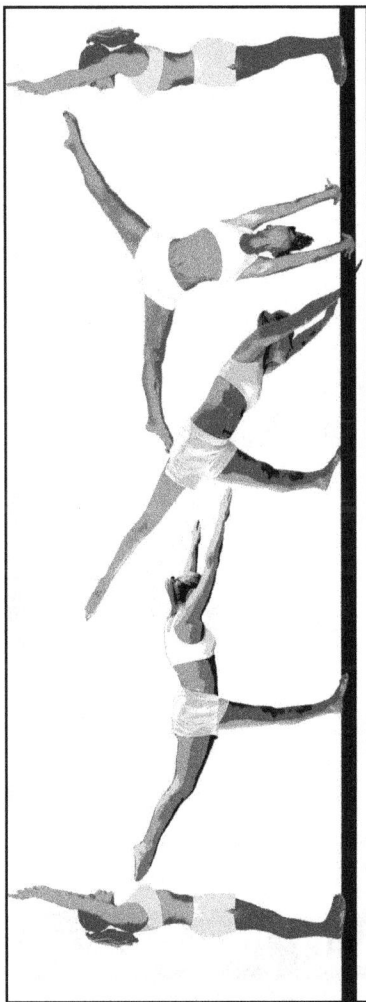

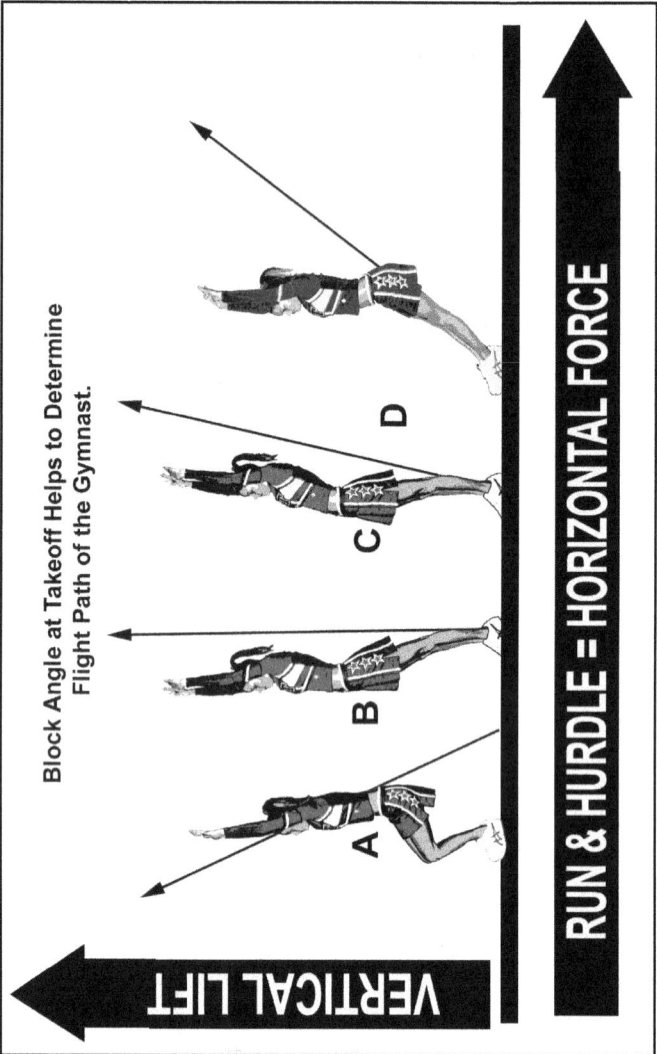

Block Angle at Takeoff Helps to Determine Flight Path of the Gymnast.

A   B   C   D

VERTICAL LIFT

RUN & HURDLE = HORIZONTAL FORCE

Importance of the Round Off

The round off is the transitional skill (transfers power from one element to another) from the run and hurdle to back handsprings, somersaults, and several other skills. Yet, even with this all-important role the round off is easily one of the most neglected skills from a coaching standpoint.

The position of your body at the end of the snap down from the round off is crucial to the setup of the following skill. If you land with your feet in the "A" position (see illustration page 30), which is typical for many novice tumblers, you will most likely have little or no power for the next tumbling skill. If you are doing a back handspring from this position, you will most likely buckle your knees on takeoff or gain forward (cause your body to move forward rather than backward) which is not a good takeoff position for back handsprings or any other tumbling skill.

The only way for you to get into a back handspring from the "A" position is to buckle (bend) your knees so you can get your center of gravity past the vertical position, which will allow you to travel backwards but will drastically reduce the power of the skill.

If you snap down with your feet closer to the "B" position, you will certainly transfer more power from the run and hurdle with nice tight legs and good stretch of the upper body, but you will tend to block upward with very little rotation of your body backward. *(At more advanced levels of tumbling, this position may be appropriate for setting somersaulting skills.)*

Moving into a back handspring from block angle "C" can still be a little scary. Although you may land straight up and down on the floor from the snap down of your round off, the horizontal force from takeoff or more forcefully from a hurdle and round off will cause your body to continue rotating backward – just a bit higher in the air than is normally recommended for a competent back handspring.

"B" and to some degree "C" are standard takeoff positions for back somersaults. "C" is typical for novice gymnasts learning back tuck somersaults, although not necessarily ideal. "B" is a good position for setting layout somersaults when combined with a strong horizontal force from the run, hurdle, and round off or a takeoff from a similar position from a back handspring.

Always focus on SAFETY!

Block angle "D" would likely be the ideal takeoff position into the back handspring with straight, tight legs punching through the floor.

The following drills emphasize the landing positions needed for training the rebound and for training the transition from round off to the back handspring.

Drill: Round off rebound

Special Note: This is a skill that falls into the "good to demonstrate one aspect of a technique, but not-so-good for the overall skill" category. The one aspect to get is a clean jump-hurdle to front-side-back style round off. (This is good training for a round off into a back tuck somersault.)

Purpose: To teach you that correct technique for a front-side-back round off may be initiated from a stand rather than from an out of control run across the floor.

Directions: Jump from two feet to a hurdle and focus on entering this skill as though you are about to kick up to a handstand. When your hands are inches from the floor, pivot ¼ turn, and then pivot another ¼ turn at the handstand before squaring your hips to snap down, by blocking off the floor through your shoulders and chest to a hollow position.

In this instance, you do want to execute a controlled rebound that shows some amplitude, so snap down and land with your feet behind your body in position "B" *(see page 30).* The key is in lifting your head and chest quickly from the snap down so you are spotting something at eye level, which will help you to control your balance when landing from the rebound.

Note: This should be a rebound (punch off the floor) and not a bent knee jump into the rebound position.

Spotting/Safety Tip: The chance for over-rotation on the rebound is high for athletes new to this skill. Ask a qualified coach to spot you for possible over-rotation. Review safety landing drills, especially the backwards landing with "rock and roll" technique before practicing this skill on the floor exercise mat.

Round off rebound

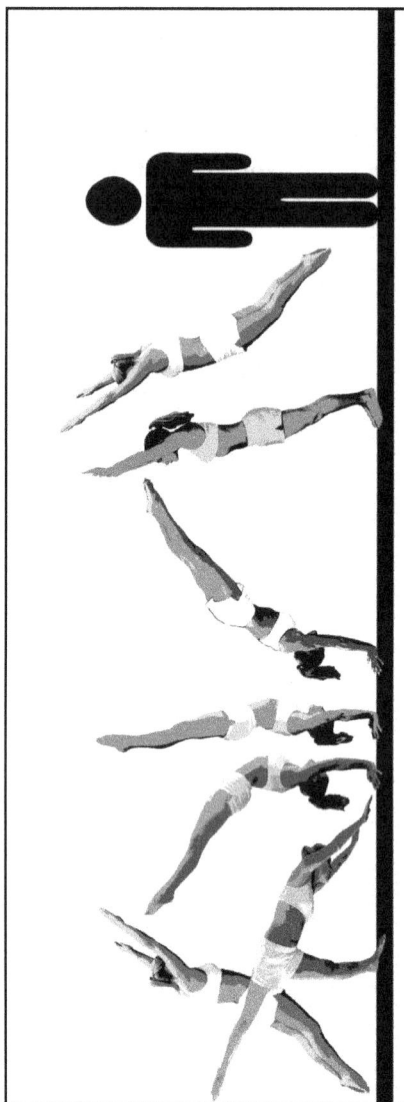

Drill: [From stretch position] One leg at horizontal; drive into F-S-B round off with rebound to stick position.

Purpose: Similar to the last drill, but instead of a jump to a hurdle, you must now refine the technique even more to do it correctly. Running and jumping should not be a substitute for correct technique.

Directions: From a standing stretch position, you will lift one leg slightly above horizontal and then take a large step forward, driving the upper body down to the ground to initiate a front-side-back round off with a rebound to a stick landing position.

Note: Start this drill on a line on the floor to give yourself feedback about how straight you are tumbling. If you land off to one side or the other of the line, it is likely that you are turning too early in the front (or lead up to the handstand) portion of the round off. The lower you can drive your upper body in the handstand kick up portion of the drill, before pivoting your body sideways, the more square your body will be on the line at the finish of the skill. **Ask your coach to spot the rebound, if necessary.**

F-S-B round off with rebound to stick position

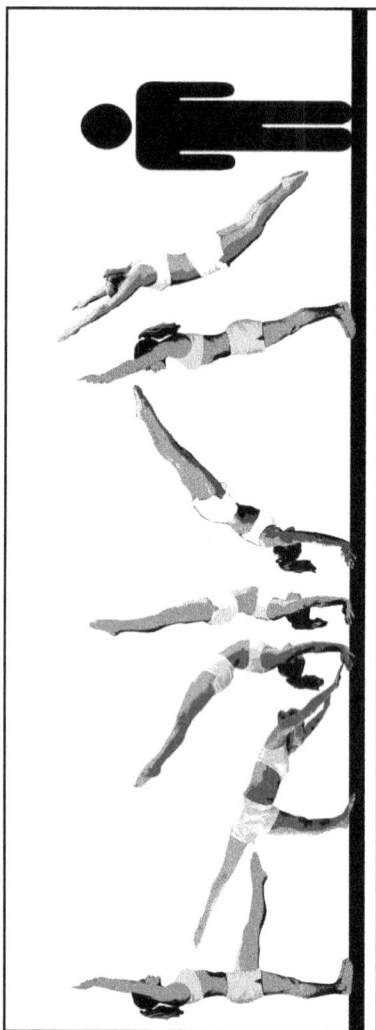

Safety Note: Hand Position

In both the handstand and the round off, it is very important that you **position your hands correctly** to prevent injury to the wrists, elbows, and arms. If your **hands** are **turned out,** you can cause the elbows to lock which **could lead to hyperextension injuries, dislocations, or worse.** One safe way to place your hands on the floor during a handstand or round off is:

1. Put your arms straight out in front of you, shoulder-width apart, with your palms facing toward the floor with all your fingers pointing forward.

2. With your palms still facing toward the floor stick your thumbs out to the side and slowly bring your arms together until the tips of your thumbs are touching each other.

3. Now, extend both wrists upward so your fingers point toward the ceiling.

4. With thumbs touching and fingers pointing toward the ceiling, rotate your hands until the index fingers on both hands are almost touching. Done correctly, you will notice that you have created a somewhat triangular space between your thumbs and index fingers (see Figure 1).

Always focus on SAFETY!

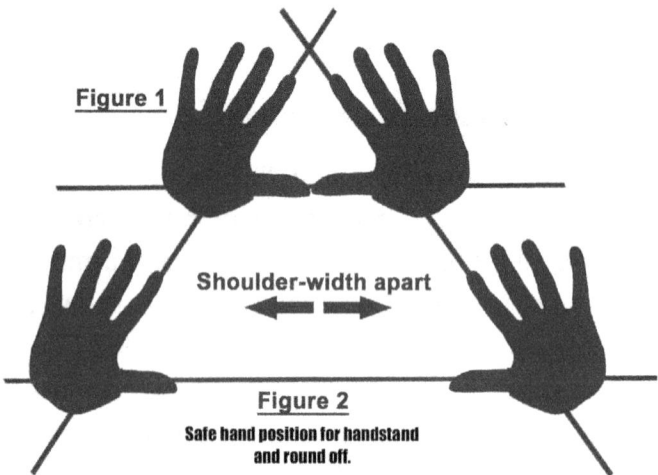

Figure 1

Shoulder-width apart

Figure 2

Safe hand position for handstand
and round off.

5. Keeping your hands in this slightly turned in position, separate your arms again until they are shoulder-width apart (see Figure 2). This is an appropriate hand placement on the floor for handstands and round offs (even back handsprings) – of course, your arms will be up next to your ears and not in front of your body when performing the skill.

Note: Advanced level tumblers may be coached to a different hand placement on the round off, however, until you have mastered the fundamentals, stick with a safe hand placement.

Chicken tracking

I have no idea where the name for this technique came from – but it is useful and visual.

Before doing a tumbling pass, like a round off back handspring, grab a piece of chalk from bars and liberally coat your hands.

Perform your tumbling pass as normal, then go back and study the marks you left on the floor.

Study your hand placement.

Study your alignment on the tumbling pass.

Does the first hand leave drag marks from your fingers? This happens when you push off your front leg too early.

Does the second hand barely leave a mark? You may be pivoting primarily on the first hand and getting little help from the second hand.

Don't forget to clean the mess you made before moving to your next event.

Summary

Once again, thanks for buying my book and getting all the way to the end.

I hope you will find these techniques useful and they improve your gymnastics skills.

Please keep in mind the techniques presented here are for a fictitious (made up) gymnast. That means they may not work as effectively for you unless they have been adapted to your skill, conditioning, and technical abilities by a qualified gymnastics coach.

Remember, **always focus on safety!**

For more information about the round off, especially how to effectively connect it to the back handspring or use it as a set up for a back tuck, get your copy of **"Back Handsprings: The Secret Techniques,"** available at bookstores online.

Amazon: https://amzn.to/3qW4lFY

Barnes & Noble: https://bit.ly/37ZOMEO

For more information contact:

Richardson Publishing

PO Box 162115

Altamonte Springs, FL 32716

coachrik@aol.com

www.ingramcontent.com/pod-product-compliance
Lightning Source LLC
Chambersburg PA
CBHW071938020426
42331CB00010B/2929